GUIDE SEVEN:
ROOTED TOGETHER
*From Root to Tip: A Growing Hands
Guide for Natural Hair*

BY CONSTANCE HUNTER

For permissions, inquiries, or additional resources, please contact:

Pre'Vail Natural Hair Salon

www.prevailyournatural.com | prevailyournatural@gmail.com

This book is intended for informational and educational purposes only and should serve as a general guide to understanding and improving natural hair health. While the methods and recommendations provided are based on expertise in natural hair care and trichology, they are not intended to replace professional medical or dermatological advice.

If you are experiencing severe scalp conditions, excessive hair loss, or other persistent issues, it is strongly recommended that you consult a licensed dermatologist or a professional cosmetologist specializing in scalp and hair health. A trained professional can assess underlying causes and provide personalized treatment plans tailored to your specific needs.

By using the information in this book, the reader acknowledges that the author and publisher are not responsible for individual outcomes. Readers should exercise their own discretion when applying the suggested practices.

First Edition: 2025

ISBN:

Paperback: 978-1-968134-07-5

Ebook: 978-1-968134-16-7

Printed in USA

ABOUT THE AUTHOR

As a certified trichologist and natural hair care educator, I specialize in helping individuals discover what's truly possible for their hair—especially when they've been told otherwise.

My passion lies in witnessing transformation—that moment when someone realizes their hair can be healthy, strong, and free. With a deep understanding of the science behind hair and scalp health, I strive to provide clarity, comfort, and actionable solutions. My training equips me to assess and guide care for a wide range of concerns, from common challenges like dandruff and dryness to complex conditions such as alopecia areata, scalp psoriasis, and CCCA.

But my work goes beyond diagnosis or technique. I believe in education, empowerment, and helping clients build routines that nourish their crown from root to tip. This includes learning to read labels, choosing products with purpose, avoiding harmful styling practices, and embracing care that fits their lifestyle and values.

While I offer expert insight from the field of trichology, I'm not a medical doctor. Hair and scalp symptoms can sometimes signal deeper health issues. That's why I encourage a holistic approach—and, when necessary, consulting licensed healthcare professionals for comprehensive support.

In this series, you'll find guidance rooted in science, experience, and care. My hope is that it not only helps you understand your hair better but also love it more, trust it more, and grow with it in ways you never thought possible.

Your hair is not the problem—you just needed the right guide.

DEDICATION

For those who thought they had to do this alone,
You're not the only one. And you never were.

OVERVIEW

You don't have to walk this journey alone. *Rooted Together* explores the power of community, representation, and shared experience in natural hair care. From workplace confidence to cultural pride, this guide helps you find support—and be support—on the path to wholeness.

Healthy hair is personal, but it's also political. And sometimes, the best thing for your hair isn't a product—it's people.

SERIES INTRODUCTION

Welcome to *From Root to Tip: A Growing Hands Guide for Natural Hair*

This series was created with one goal in mind: to give you what's been missing—not just products, not just trends, but truth, support, and real guidance for real people who are ready to finally understand and care for their natural hair from the inside out.

For years, we've been taught to manage, fix, or fight our hair. But here, we're doing something different. We're returning to care—not control. To confidence. To consistency. To choice.

Each guide in this series is built as a step in your journey. They can be read in order or on their own, depending on where you are in your process. Whether you're just starting out, rebuilding your relationship with your hair, or deepening your understanding, this space is for you.

I've written these guides from my hands—growing hands that have touched, healed, protected, and restored countless crowns. Now, I offer that care to you.

This isn't just about hair. It's about healing. It's about reclaiming your rhythm, your confidence, and your beauty—from root to tip.

Let's begin.

WHAT YOU WILL LEARN

- How to find and join natural hair communities (online and in person)

- Navigating workplace policies, bias, and conversations with confidence

- The impact of representation in schools, media, and salons

- How to use your hair story to inspire others

- Advocacy tips for creating safer, more inclusive spaces

- Understanding hair as an extension of identity and culture

WHAT YOU'LL WALK AWAY WITH

- A deeper connection to the cultural and communal power of natural hair

- The confidence to stand tall in your truth—anywhere

- Tools to build, lead, or support safe spaces for others

- A renewed sense of pride in being part of a bigger movement

TABLE OF CONTENTS

INTRODUCTION

Your hair is a story—and every story needs a space to be told.

In *Rooted Together*, we dive into what it means to belong while embracing your natural hair. We talk about showing up confidently in professional spaces, connecting with others on similar journeys, and using your voice to advocate for acceptance, visibility, and self-expression.

This guide reminds you that your crown is part of something bigger. It honors the history behind your hair, the community that surrounds it, and the legacy you're helping shape every time you show up as yourself.

LESSON 1:
FINDING AND JOINING NATURAL HAIR COMMUNITIES

Locating and Becoming a Part of Local and Online Communities

Navigating the world of natural hair can be a transformative journey, and one of the most valuable aspects of this experience is connecting with others who share similar interests and goals. Sharing experiences, tips, and encouragement with others can provide motivation, accountability, and valuable insights. Building a community around hair care and wellness not only fosters a sense of belonging but also helps you achieve your goals more effectively. Here's how to build and benefit from a supportive community.

Finding Like-Minded Individuals

1. **Local Groups and Meetups**

Local communities offer a sense of belonging and direct support. Start by researching natural hair meetups, workshops, or events in your area. Websites like Meetup.com, Eventbrite, or local community boards can help you find gatherings focused on natural hair care and styling. Look for events, workshops, or clubs that focus on hair care, wellness, or beauty. These gatherings provide opportunities to learn from others, try new products or techniques, and build friendships. Engaging with fellow naturals in person fosters deeper connections and allows for direct support.

2. **Professional Networks**

Connecting with professionals in the hair care and wellness industry, such as hairstylists, trichologists, and wellness coaches, can provide expert advice and guidance.

Attend industry events, follow professionals on social media, and participate in webinars or workshops to expand your network.

3. Online Communities

Social media is a powerful tool for locating both local and global natural hair communities. Online groups, forums, and websites dedicated to hair care provide spaces to exchange tips, product recommendations, and personal experiences. Platforms like Instagram, Facebook, and Reddit host vibrant communities focused on natural hair care, wellness, and self-care.

Engaging with online communities can provide a sense of belonging, especially for those in areas with fewer resources.

4. Attend Natural Hair Festivals and Expos

Natural hair festivals and expos are important events where you can meet others passionate about natural hair. These events often feature vendors, workshops, and panels covering a range of topics related to natural hair care. Attending these events offers opportunities to network with fellow attendees and industry professionals, learn about the latest trends, and gain valuable insights into natural hair care.

5. Engage with Online Forums and Groups

Numerous online forums and discussion boards serve as gathering places for natural hair enthusiasts to share experiences and advice. Websites like Reddit, Naturally Curly, and Hair Care Forum have active communities discussing various aspects of natural hair care. Participate in these forums by asking questions, sharing your experiences, and joining discussions to build connections and expand your knowledge.

Benefits of Connecting with Others on a Natural Hair Journey

1. Access to Knowledge and Expertise

Communities often serve as repositories of valuable knowledge, where members share tips, product recommendations, and techniques that have worked for them. Whether you're looking for advice on a specific hair concern or seeking fresh styling ideas, the collective wisdom of these communities can be an invaluable resource.

- **Personal Stories:** Sharing your hair care journey and wellness experiences can inspire and support others facing similar challenges. Personal stories offer relatable insights and practical advice. Whether through blog posts, social media updates, or group discussions, your experiences can be a valuable resource for others.

- **Tips and Tricks:** Exchange practical tips and tricks within your community. Whether it's a new hair care technique, a product that worked wonders, or a wellness practice that improved your life, sharing these nuggets of wisdom can help others on their journey. Be open to receiving advice as well—your community's collective knowledge can be an enriching source of information.

- **Product Recommendations:** Discussing products that have worked for you and learning about others' favorites can help you discover new solutions. Honest reviews and recommendations guide you in choosing the best products for your hair type and wellness needs, saving both time and money.

2. Emotional Support and Encouragement

Embracing natural hair can come with its challenges, and having a supportive network can make all the difference. In a community of support, you'll find the encouragement and motivation to stay committed to your hair care and wellness journey. Every success, no matter how small, deserves celebration, and kind words can lift your spirits during challenging moments. When others believe in your goals, your confidence and dedication soar. Hair care and wellness aren't always easy—they can test your patience and emotions. But in a community, you discover a safe haven where frustrations are shared, advice flows freely, and emotional support is always within reach. There's comfort in knowing you're not alone on this path. Drawing inspiration from the victories and perseverance of others empowers you to keep pushing forward, and in return, you can offer that same encouragement to others. Witnessing others triumph serves as a reminder that you, too, can overcome any challenge. Together, we rise.

3. Exposure to Diverse Perspectives

Natural hair communities are diverse and inclusive, offering a variety of perspectives and experiences. Engaging with people from different backgrounds and hair types can broaden your understanding of natural hair care and styling. This exposure helps you discover new methods and approaches that may resonate with your unique hair needs. When seeking a community to support your hair care and wellness journey, look for these essential qualities:

- **Respect and Kindness:** A truly empowering group is built on respect and kindness. Choose a community that values open, non-judgmental communication, where every voice is heard and appreciated. In this space, differing opinions and experiences are respected, and negativity or criticism has no place.

- **Inclusivity:** The best communities welcome everyone with open arms, regardless of hair type, background, or experience level. Diversity is celebrated, and each member is encouraged to share their unique perspectives and traditions. This inclusivity enriches the group and deepens everyone's understanding and appreciation for each other's journeys.

In a group that upholds these values, you'll find the support, inspiration, and empowerment to thrive on your personal journey.

4. Opportunities for Learning and Growth

Being part of a community offers continuous opportunities for learning and personal growth. Growth thrives in environments that prioritize learning. Seek a community that stays informed about the latest in hair care, wellness, products, and techniques. Whether through shared resources, educational content, or guest experts, a focus on continuous learning keeps the community vibrant, knowledgeable, and inspired.

5. Building Lasting Connections

Building lasting connections with others who share your passion for natural hair can lead to meaningful relationships. These connections can become sources of friendship, collaboration, and support. Whether you connect with someone locally or online, forming these relationships enriches your natural hair journey and provides a strong sense of community.

6. Inspiration and Motivation

Connecting with others in natural hair communities can be a significant source of inspiration and motivation. Seeing how others style their hair, maintain their routines, and overcome challenges can inspire you to try new techniques and stay committed to your own hair care goals. Having a community that holds you accountable can help you stay on track with your routines. Sharing your objectives and progress with others creates a sense of responsibility. Regular check-ins, whether online or in person, can keep you focused and motivated.

Celebrating others' successes and sharing your own achievements fosters a positive and motivating environment.

In summary, finding and joining natural hair communities can greatly enhance your hair journey. Whether through local groups, online platforms, or industry events, connecting with others provides access to valuable knowledge, emotional support, diverse perspectives, and opportunities for personal growth. By actively participating in these communities, you can build lasting relationships, gain inspiration, and stay motivated as you embrace and celebrate your natural hair. The support, knowledge, and inspiration gained from these communities are invaluable, helping you navigate your hair journey with confidence and joy. Embrace the sense of belonging and the wealth of shared experiences that come from being part of a natural hair community.

LESSON 2:
EMBRACING NATURAL HAIR IN THE WORKPLACE

Embracing your natural hair in a professional setting can be empowering, but it also presents unique challenges. Many individuals grapple with maintaining a polished, professional appearance while showcasing their natural texture. Overcoming workplace biases and stereotypes is entirely achievable with the right approach. Here are some tips to help you confidently showcase your natural hair at work while maintaining a polished and professional image.

Tips for Maintaining a Professional Appearance While Embracing Natural Hair

1. Understand Your Company's Dress Code and Culture

Consider your workplace culture and dress code. While some environments are more conservative, others are more relaxed and accepting of diverse styles. Many organizations have revised their policies to be more inclusive, but it's important to understand your company's specific expectations. Being familiar with your workplace culture allows you to choose hairstyles that align with professional standards while staying true to your natural hair.

2. Invest in Professional-Quality Hair Care Products

To ensure your natural hair looks polished and professional, invest in high-quality hair care products designed for your hair type. Look for products that promote the health and appearance of your hair, such as moisturizing shampoos, conditioners, and styling creams. Consistently using these products will help you achieve a neat, well-groomed look that exudes professionalism.

3. Opt for Well-Kept, Defined Styles

Natural hair offers a wide range of versatile styling options suitable for professional settings. Focus on hairstyles that are defined, well-maintained, and polished.

Some popular options include:

- **Buns:** Sleek, high or low buns are timeless, elegant, and professional.

- **Twist-Outs and Braid-Outs:** These styles create defined curls that can be styled neatly. Puffs and Ponytails: A well-groomed puff or ponytail looks chic and work-appropriate.

- **Protective Styles:** Braids, twists, and updos not only protect your hair but also projects a polished image.

Regular maintenance, such as trimming, detangling, and moisturizing, is key to keeping your natural hair looking its best.

4. Use Accessories Wisely

Hair accessories can elevate your natural hairstyle while maintaining a polished, professional look. Opt for accessories that enhance your style and add a touch of sophistication. Headbands, hairpins, and scarves can not only complement your outfit but also keep your hair neat and tidy. Choose subtle accessories that align with your professional attire.

5. Confidence and Poise

Confidence is everything. Embrace your natural hair with pride, as it communicates a powerful and positive message to your colleagues. Stand tall, smile, and engage with others self-assuredly, allowing your professionalism to shine through effortlessly.

6. Seek Inspiration from Professionals

Take inspiration from professionals who wear natural hair confidently in their workplaces. Many public figures, entrepreneurs, and influencers successfully balance their careers with natural hairstyles. Observing how they style their hair can spark ideas and boost your confidence in presenting your own natural hair professionally.

Overcoming Workplace Biases and Stereotypes

1. Educate and Advocate

Biases often arise from a lack of understanding. Take opportunities to educate your colleagues about natural hair, highlighting its versatility and cultural significance. Sharing this information can help dispel myths and contribute to fostering a more inclusive workplace.

2. Be Prepared for Questions

Colleagues might express curiosity about your hair. Responding with patience and openness can transform these moments into valuable educational opportunities. Share your hair care practices and the unique beauty of natural hair with enthusiasm.

3. Set Professional Boundaries

While educating others is important, it's equally crucial to set boundaries. If questions or comments about your hair become intrusive or inappropriate, address them politely but firmly. Communicating what is acceptable helps protect your comfort and maintain professionalism.

4. Seek Allies and Support

Identify workplace allies who champion diversity and inclusion. These individuals can offer support and assist in advocating for a more inclusive environment. Additionally, employee resource groups focused on diversity can provide a sense of community and encouragement.

5. Know Your Rights

Understand your workplace policies regarding discrimination and diversity. If you experience bias or discrimination, be aware of the proper channels to report such incidents. Knowing your rights empowers you to act confidently when necessary.

6. Lead by Example

Be a role model by confidently embracing your natural hair in the workplace. Your professionalism and self-assurance can inspire others to do the same, helping to shift perceptions and promote a more inclusive culture. By leading through example, you contribute to creating a more accepting and supportive environment.

7. Document Your Experiences

Keep a detailed record of any instances of bias or discrimination related to your natural hair. This documentation can be invaluable if you need to escalate the issue to HR or higher management. A well-documented account strengthens your case and ensures your concerns are addressed appropriately.

8. Promote Awareness and Inclusion

Advocate for greater awareness and inclusion in your workplace. Support or initiate efforts that celebrate diversity and educate colleagues about different hair types and styles. Organizing or participating in diversity events, workshops, and discussions can play a significant role in fostering an inclusive culture.

9. Maintain Confidence and Resilience

Dealing with workplace biases can be challenging, but your confidence and resilience are key. Your natural hair is a meaningful part of your identity and self-expression—embrace it with pride. Stay true to yourself, and remember that your authenticity adds value to the workplace, regardless of external pressures or biases.

Embracing natural hair in the workplace is a bold and empowering act of self-acceptance and cultural pride. By maintaining a polished, professional appearance with versatile hairstyles, proper maintenance, and thoughtful accessories, you can confidently showcase your natural hair. Addressing workplace biases requires educating others, setting boundaries, seeking support, and knowing your rights. With confidence and poise, you can navigate the professional world while proudly wearing your natural hair, helping to create a more inclusive and diverse workplace.

LESSON 3:
INSPIRING OTHERS TO EMBRACE THEIR NATURAL HAIR

Your natural hair journey is not just personal—it holds the power to inspire and uplift others. Advocacy and representation play a pivotal role in encouraging individuals to embrace their natural hair. By sharing your story and celebrating the beauty of natural hair, you can inspire others to confidently wear their natural locks and embrace their unique identity. Here's how you can advocate for the natural hair community and inspire others along the way:

Advocacy and Representation in the Natural Hair Community

1. Understanding the Role of Advocacy

Advocacy means actively supporting and promoting a cause. In the context of natural hair, it involves championing the beauty, diversity, and acceptance of natural textures. Advocacy is vital for challenging outdated stereotypes and combating biases that have marginalized natural hair types for generations. By advocating for natural hair, you contribute to shifting societal norms and fostering inclusivity.

2. The Impact of Representation

Representation is powerful—it shapes how individuals see themselves and their identity. When people see others who look like them celebrated and accepted, it fosters validation and belonging. In the natural hair community, representation involves showcasing diverse textures and styles across media, workplaces, and public spaces. Positive representation dismantles harmful stereotypes, empowering individuals to embrace their natural hair with confidence.

3. Becoming a Role Model

By embracing your natural hair, you can become a role model for others. Your journey can inspire those who may feel unsure or self-conscious about their texture. Confidently wearing your natural hair and sharing your experiences sends a powerful message: natural hair is not only beautiful but also a meaningful form of self-expression. Role models like you help normalize natural hair and encourage others to see it as professional, versatile, and celebrated.

4. Advocating for Inclusive Policies

Advocacy extends to driving policy changes that promote natural hair acceptance. Grooming policies in workplaces, schools, and institutions often contain biases against natural hair. By advocating for inclusive policies, you help create environments where everyone feels respected and valued. Engage in conversations with decision-makers, participate in diversity initiatives, and support organizations championing policy reform to ensure natural hair is recognized and celebrated.

5. Building a Supportive Community

Participating in and building supportive communities amplifies advocacy efforts. Join or create groups, forums, or online spaces focused on natural hair. These platforms allow individuals to share experiences, exchange tips, and provide encouragement. By contributing to these communities, you strengthen a collective effort to uplift and celebrate natural hair, fostering a sense of connection and shared purpose.

Sharing Your Journey to Inspire Others

1. Reflecting on Your Personal Journey

Sharing your natural hair journey begins with reflecting on your experiences—the challenges and triumphs you've encountered along the way. Think about how your relationship with your natural hair has evolved and the factors that shaped your current perspective.

Revisit moments of self-discovery, growth, and learning, and consider how they've influenced your understanding of natural beauty. Be candid about struggles with self-acceptance, societal pressures, and the path to embracing your natural hair. Your openness can resonate deeply with others facing similar experiences, offering them encouragement and hope.

2. Highlighting Key Milestones

Identify significant milestones in your natural hair journey. These might include the moment you first embraced your natural texture, overcame a particular challenge, or achieved a personal hair care goal. Sharing these milestones creates a roadmap for others, showing that progress and transformation are achievable. Each milestone reflects a step forward, offering inspiration to those on their own journeys.

3. Sharing Challenges and Solutions

Be transparent about the challenges you've faced and the solutions you've discovered. Discuss topics like societal pressures, self-doubt, or managing hair care routines. Sharing practical advice and strategies can be invaluable for those navigating similar situations.

Talk about your favorite products, styling techniques, and hair care practices, offering tips to simplify the transition to natural hair. By being honest about both the highs and lows, your story becomes relatable and authentic, inspiring others while equipping them with actionable insights.

4. Using Social Media and Other Platforms

Social media and other platforms offer a powerful way to share your natural hair journey with a broader audience. Create content such as blog posts, videos, or social media updates that showcase your experiences. Share tips, tutorials, and personal stories to inspire and educate others. By leveraging these platforms, you can connect with a diverse audience and spread messages of empowerment and acceptance.

5. Hosting Workshops and Events

Organize workshops or events centered around natural hair. These can include hair care tutorials, self-esteem workshops, or panel discussions on the cultural significance of natural hair. Such events create opportunities to engage directly with others, share valuable information, and foster meaningful dialogue. They also help build a sense of community and support for individuals embracing their natural hair.

6. Collaborating with Influencers and Organizations

Partner with influencers, brands, and organizations that align with your advocacy goals. Collaborations can amplify your message and broaden your reach. Joint social media campaigns, guest appearances on podcasts or blogs, or co-hosting events are great ways to work together. These partnerships strengthen your impact and promote a more inclusive narrative around natural hair.

7. Encouraging Self-Love and Acceptance

Inspiring others to embrace their natural hair starts with promoting self-love and acceptance. Encourage individuals to view their natural hair as a unique and valuable part of their identity. Share affirmations and messages that highlight the beauty and strength of natural hair. By fostering positivity and self-acceptance, you empower others to embrace their natural beauty with confidence.

8. Celebrating Success Stories

Highlight the success stories of individuals who have embraced their natural hair and experienced transformative changes in their lives. These testimonials serve as powerful examples of the benefits of embracing natural hair. By showcasing diverse experiences and achievements, you reinforce the idea that natural hair is a source of pride and confidence.

9. Embracing Continuous Growth and Learning

Encourage a mindset of ongoing growth and learning. Share resources, books, or guides that have supported you in your natural hair journey. Promoting continuous education and self- discovery helps others embrace and celebrate their natural beauty. By staying informed and open to new ideas, you contribute to a culture of empowerment and support within the natural hair community.

Inspiring others to embrace their natural hair involves a multifaceted approach that blends advocacy, representation, and personal storytelling. By advocating for natural hair acceptance, sharing your journey, and offering practical advice, you contribute to a more inclusive and empowering narrative. Through these efforts, you help others recognize and celebrate their natural beauty, fostering a community rooted in confidence and pride.

LESSON 4:
HAIR AS A SYMBOL OF IDENTITY

Hair is more than just a physical attribute; it is a profound symbol of identity and self- expression. For many, especially within the natural hair community, hair embodies cultural heritage, personal history, and individuality. This lesson explores the deep cultural and personal significance of natural hair, examining how it serves as a symbol of identity and how to navigate conversations about identity and self-expression through hair.

Exploring the Cultural and Personal Significance of Natural Hair

1. Cultural Heritage and Identity

Natural hair often serves as a powerful expression of cultural heritage. For many communities, particularly those of African descent, natural hair is a tangible link to ancestral traditions and values. Historically, natural hair textures and styles were significant markers of identity and community. Traditional hairstyles, such as braids, twists, and afros, were not only aesthetic choices but also carried cultural meanings, signifying social status, rites of passage, and communal affiliations.

In modern contexts, embracing natural hair can be an act of reclaiming cultural pride and resisting historical and ongoing discrimination. For many, wearing their hair naturally is a way to honor their heritage and challenge societal norms that have long marginalized or invalidated natural textures.

2. Personal Expression and Self-Identity

On a personal level, natural hair is a form of self-expression, allowing individuals to showcase their unique identity and personality. Hairstyles can be a canvas for creativity, reflecting one's mood, style, and preferences. For many, the journey to embracing natural hair is intertwined with a broader journey of self-discovery and self-acceptance. As individuals learn to love and care for their natural hair, they often experience a profound sense of empowerment and confidence.

Natural hair can also represent a personal rebellion against societal beauty standards. By choosing to wear their hair naturally, individuals assert their right to define beauty on their own terms, rejecting pressure to conform to mainstream ideals that may not resonate with their personal identity. Natural hair represents strength, resilience, and the ongoing fight for equality and representation.

3. Intersection of Identity and Hair

The intersection of identity and hair is complex, encompassing factors such as race, gender, and personal experiences. For people of color, natural hair is often a significant aspect of their racial and cultural identity. Hair texture and styling choices may reflect a desire to connect with—or distance oneself from—certain cultural or societal expectations.

In discussions about gender identity, natural hair also plays a role. Non-binary and genderqueer individuals, for example, may use hairstyles as a means of expressing their gender identity and challenging traditional gender norms. Hair can be a powerful tool for articulating and visualizing one's gender expression, fostering connections with others who understand the significance of the natural hair journey. Celebrating natural hair within a community provides support, encouragement, and a sense of belonging.

4. Navigating Conversations About Identity and Self-Expression

▪ Understanding the Complexity of Identity

When navigating conversations about natural hair, it is important to recognize the complexity of identity. Hair is deeply personal, and its significance varies widely among individuals.

Approach discussions with sensitivity and an openness to diverse perspectives.

Each person's relationship with their hair is shaped by cultural, social, and personal factors. Educating others about the rich traditions and meanings behind natural hairstyles fosters understanding and appreciation. Sharing knowledge and experiences can help challenge misconceptions and promote inclusivity

▪ Respecting Personal Choices

Respecting individual choices about hair is crucial. Whether someone chooses to wear their hair naturally, straightened, or styled in a particular way, it is important to honor their decision and the reasons behind it. Avoid making assumptions or judgments based on hair appearance, recognizing that its significance is deeply personal and unique.

▪ Addressing Hair Discrimination

Conversations about natural hair often intersect with discussions about discrimination and bias. Many individuals face prejudice and professional or social pressures related to their hair.

Address these issues with empathy and support, advocating for greater acceptance and inclusivity. Understanding the historical and ongoing challenges faced by people with natural hair can help create more respectful and supportive dialogues.

- **Educating and Raising Awareness**

Navigating conversations about natural hair involves raising awareness about its significance. Sharing information on the cultural and historical contexts of natural hair, as well as personal stories, can illustrate its importance. By fostering understanding and appreciation, you contribute to a more inclusive environment where diverse expressions of identity are celebrated.

- **Promoting Positive Representation**

Positive representation plays a key role in shaping how natural hair is perceived and valued. Advocate for greater visibility of natural hair in media, advertising, and professional settings. Support and celebrate diverse representations of natural hair that challenge stereotypes and highlight the beauty of different textures and styles.

- **Encouraging Open Dialogue**

Create spaces for open dialogue where people can share their experiences and perspectives on natural hair. Encourage conversations that explore the intersections of hair, identity, and self- expression. By providing a platform for these discussions, you help build a supportive community where individuals feel heard and valued.

- Fostering Self-Acceptance and Confidence

Encourage self-acceptance and confidence in embracing natural hair. Share strategies and resources for hair care and styling that promote healthy hair and boost self-esteem. Supporting individuals in their journey toward self-love and acceptance helps foster a positive and empowering environment.

- **Supporting Personal Growth**

Support personal growth and exploration in the context of hair and identity. Encourage individuals to experiment with different styles and discover what feels authentic to them. Recognize that the journey to embracing natural hair is often a process of self-discovery and personal growth.

- **Building Community and Solidarity**

Foster a sense of community and solidarity among those who embrace natural hair. Connecting with others who share similar experiences and values can create a network of support and encouragement, helping individuals navigate their personal journeys with natural hair.

In summary, serves as a powerful symbol of identity and self-expression, deeply rooted in cultural heritage and personal experience. Navigating conversations about natural hair requires understanding its complexity, respecting individual choices, and advocating for greater acceptance and representation.

By fostering open dialogue, promoting positive representation, and supporting personal growth, we can help create a more inclusive and empowering environment for embracing natural hair. The journey of embracing natural hair is one of self-discovery and empowerment—one that reflects the beauty and diversity of human identity.

QUIZ
BUILDING A SUPPORTIVE COMMUNITY

Lesson 1: Finding and Joining Natural Hair Communities

1. Question

What is one way to find natural hair communities?

a) Only attending professional hair shows.

b) Searching for online forums, social media groups, and local events dedicated to natural hair.

c) Asking only professional hairstylists for recommendations.

d) Visiting salons that only cater to chemically treated hair.

Answer: b) Searching for online forums, social media groups, and local events dedicated to natural hair.

2. Question

What is a key benefit of connecting with others on a natural hair journey?

a) Receiving free products.

b) Gaining support, advice, and encouragement from people with similar experiences.

c) Learning how to use heat styling tools.

d) Avoiding social gatherings related to hair care.

Answer: b) Gaining support, advice, and encouragement from people with similar experiences.

3. Question

How can local natural hair communities help individuals on their journey?

a) They provide an opportunity to discuss personal experiences and attend in-person workshops or events.

b) They only focus on buying expensive hair products.

c) They discourage any DIY treatments.

d) They promote chemically straightening natural hair.

Answer: a) They provide an opportunity to discuss personal experiences and attend in-person workshops or events.

Lesson 2: Embracing Natural Hair in the Workplace

1. Question

What is a tip for maintaining a professional appearance while embracing natural hair?

a) Always wear your hair straight.

b) Use styles like twists, braids, or buns that maintain a polished and neat appearance.

c) Avoid any natural hairstyles and opt for wigs.

d) Avoid washing your hair frequently.

Answer: b) Use protective styles like twists, braids, or buns that maintain a polished and neat appearance.

2. Question

What is a common workplace bias related to natural hair?

a) Natural hair is seen as unprofessional or untidy.

b) Straight hair is the only acceptable look.

c) Natural hair requires fewer products.

d) All hairstyles are accepted equally.

Answer: a) Natural hair is seen as unprofessional or untidy.

3. Question

How can individuals overcome workplace biases related to natural hair?

a) By avoiding talking about their hair journey.

b) By staying informed about workplace policies and advocating for inclusivity.

c) By wearing wigs at all times.

d) By never discussing hair in the workplace.

Answer: b) By staying informed about workplace policies and advocating for inclusivity.

Lesson 3: Inspiring Others to Embrace Their Natural Hair

1. Question

How can you inspire others to embrace their natural hair?

a) By sharing your personal hair journey and offering support to those transitioning to natural hair.

b) By discouraging others from trying new products.

c) By telling others to avoid natural hair communities.

d) By keeping your hair journey private.

Answer: a) By sharing your personal hair journey and offering support to those transitioning to natural hair.

2. Question

What role does advocacy play in the natural hair community?

a) It encourages people to avoid discussing natural hair.

b) It promotes positive representation and fights against negative stereotypes in society.

c) It discourages natural hair events and movements.

d) It focuses on eliminating natural hair styles from the workplace.

Answer: b) It promotes positive representation and fights against negative stereotypes in society.

Lesson 4: Hair as a Symbol of Identity

1. Question

Why is natural hair considered a symbol of identity?

a) It is only important for styling trends.

b) It reflects cultural heritage, personal expression, and empowerment.

c) It is not relevant to cultural or personal identity.

d) It is solely a fashion statement.

Answer: b) It reflects cultural heritage, personal expression, and empowerment.

2. Question

What is the significance of natural hair in many cultures?

a) It is purely for cosmetic purposes.

b) It holds deep cultural, historical, and personal meaning as a reflection of identity and pride.

c) It is always associated with negative stereotypes.

d) It has no significance beyond styling.

Answer: b) It holds deep cultural, historical, and personal meaning as a reflection of identity and pride.

CLOSING NOTE

You were never meant to figure this out alone.
We're stronger when we're rooted together—and your
crown connects you to something beautiful, bold, and
bigger than hair.